YOUR KNOWLEDGE HAS VALUE

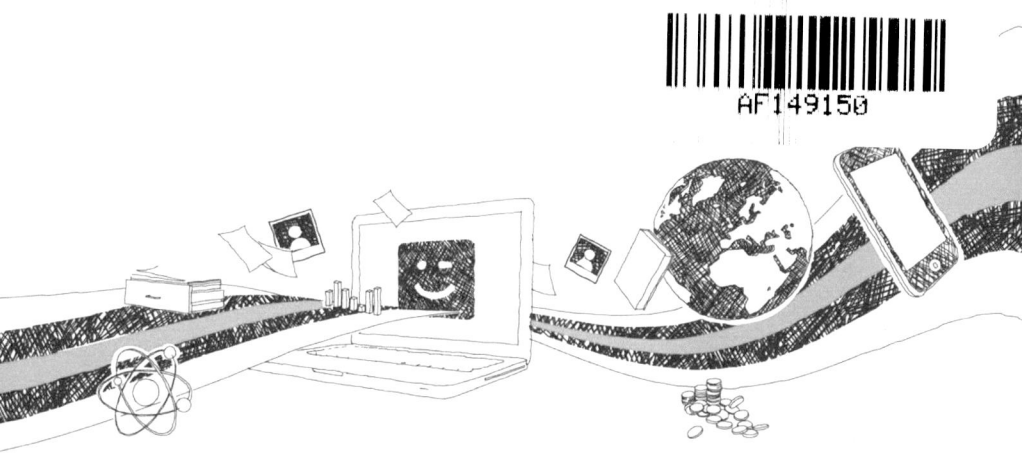

Bibliographic information published by the German National Library:

The German National Library lists this publication in the National Bibliography; detailed bibliographic data are available on the Internet at http://dnb.dnb.de .

Imprint:

Copyright © 2009 GRIN Verlag
Print and binding: Books on Demand GmbH, Norderstedt Germany
ISBN: 9783640747405

This book at GRIN:

https://www.grin.com/document/158436

Eyo Essien, Edem Williams

E-Health Services in Rural Communities of developing Countries

GRIN Verlag

GRIN - Your knowledge has value

Since its foundation in 1998, GRIN has specialized in publishing academic texts by students, college teachers and other academics as e-book and printed book. The website www.grin.com is an ideal platform for presenting term papers, final papers, scientific essays, dissertations and specialist books.

Visit us on the internet:

http://www.grin.com/

http://www.facebook.com/grincom

http://www.twitter.com/grin_com

e-Health Services in Rural Communities in the developing Countries

Essien, Eyo E. and Williams, Edem E.

Dept. Of Math/Stat & Computer Science, University of Calabar

Abstract

Health service delivery to rural communities has always been a vexed problem for most governments in developing countries. Several factors impeding the success of government programmes in this sub-sector include corruption, inadequate supply of drugs, paucity and/poor quality of medical personnel, lack of medical equipment and facilities, cost (transportation to the hospital, medical bills) to the patients of obtaining medical attention and interference by unorthodox medical practitioners. This paper surveys the problems that inhibit provision of adequate preventive and curative health care to rural communities and suggests affordable and sustainable ways in which ICT can be used to solve these problems. Special emphasis is given to use of ICT for public enlightenment for preventive health care and also for the implementation of affordable access to curative health care.

Keywords: ICT, Tele-clinic, Health Care, Tele-conferencing, Ambulance Service Support System

Introduction

Healthcare is the prevention, treatment, and management of illness and the preservation of mental and physical well being through the services offered by the medical, nursing, and allied health professions. Health care embraces all the goods and services designed to promote health, including "preventive, curative and palliative interventions, whether directed to individuals or to populations"

Health perspectives differ between rural and urban communities. The health perceptions of rural and urban residents significantly reflect their health-promotion behaviours, health maintenance, and illness treatment. Health care agencies, specialized services and infrastructure are usually less available to rural areas. Rural community members learn to distinguish between health impairments that can be tolerated for a period and those that will impede functioning. The poverty and long distances from health care providers influence the way those living in rural areas view health and address illness. Rural men and women of a variety of age groups have reported health as the ability to work and to perform one's usual activities. For example, rural workers have been found to tolerate pain for long periods and not allow it to interfere with their ability to work while urban residents concentrate in the comfort and life-prolonging aspects of health.[1]

Many of the public healthcare services like Public Health Centres (PHCs) and sub-centres in rural areas are not equipped and staffed to provide quality healthcare to the rural poor. This suggests the yawning divide between rural and urban healthcare services, between the rural poor and the well off. The new developments in healthcare have not percolated to the rural areas and this is a matter of great concern. There is therefore need to explore the ways and means to bring equity in access to health professionals and institutions between rural and urban areas.

Electronic health (e-health) describes the application of ICT across a whole range of functions that affect the healthcare industry when it comes to matters relating to health through the various solutions that exists[2]. E-health can also be described as any electronic exchange of health related data through an electronic connectivity for improving efficiency and effectiveness of health care delivery.[3] The solutions that are provided through e-health initiatives within hospitals include Hospital Management Information Systems (HMIS), telemedicine services and Internet services.

Health Management Information System
The functions of a health information system are to monitor, inform and evaluate a health system and to make clinical and management decisions.[4] Reliable and timely information on disease-specific treatment burdens within a health system is critical for the planning and monitoring of service provision. Health management information systems exist to address this need at national scales across Africa but are failing to deliver adequate data because of widespread underreporting by health facilities. Faced with this inadequacy, vital public health decisions often rely on crudely adjusted regional and national estimates of treatment burdens.[5]

Internet
There were days when patients relied on physicians for all the information concerning their health. But nowadays patients are constantly on the lookout for information regarding their health on the Internet

hence by the time they arrive at the physician's offices; they already have an idea concerning the disease that is bothering them.[6,7] However the shot coming of this solution is computer illiteracy and internet unavailability.

Aims and Objectives
The main goal this research is to develop healthy and economically productive rural citizenship through facilitating affordable, reliable and high quality health information to the rural poor using ICT.
Specific Objectives of the work can be summarized as follows:
• To develop method of providing emergency healthcare to the rural poor
• To ensure safe delivery and motherhood in rural areas
• To develop a method of providing access to health information and making healthcare accessible to the poor.
• To facilitate quality medical care to the poor in remote rural villages.
• To bridge the gap of professional isolation.

Characteristics of human health conditions in rural developing countries
In this study we use Nigeria as an example of a developing country. It is our belief that what happens in Nigeria cuts across most developing countries.
There is a dearth of medical care facilities in Nigeria's rural areas. Where health care centre exists, there is often absence of drugs; and where they are available, they are usually beyond the

reach of the poor. Nigeria's mortality and morbidity rates are amongst the highest in the world, with rural areas accounting for the majority of cases.[8] Maternal and child mortality rates are particularly disturbing, accounting for the relatively low life expectancy in Nigeria.

The public healthcare in Nigerian rural areas has the following challenges:
  (a) Access to healthcare
  (b) Quality of healthcare service delivery
  (c) Cost of healthcare

a) Access to healthcare
When people become ill, low-income households in rural areas continue to use home remedies, consult traditional healers and local providers who are often outside the formal healthcare system. Men have comparatively better access than women to healthcare options at all levels due to various socio-economic and cultural factors (including their easy mobility). The bicycle is the usual means of transport in rural villages and riding a bicycle by women is not a normal practice although tolerated in some rural communities. It is also important to say that a sick man is better attended than a sick woman. Poor women are most vulnerable to diseases and ill health as they live in unhygienic conditions, carry heavy child bearing burden, place little emphasis on their own healthcare needs, and encounter severe constraints in seeking healthcare for themselves. Fig 1 compares access to healthcare in urban and rural Nigeria.

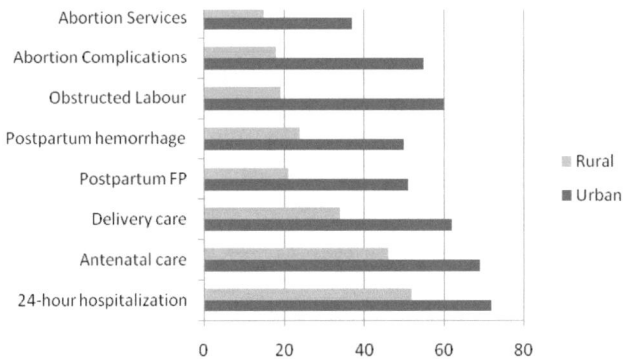

Fig 1. Comparisons of access to health services for rural and urban areas in Nigeria (source: 1995 WHO/UNICEF/UNFPA estimate of maternal mortality)

b)   Quality of healthcare service delivery

Numerous studies have indicated that the healthcare facilities at Primary Health Centre (PHC) and Sub Centre levels are mostly understaffed and short of drugs and essential supplies and that they sometimes suffer from low staff morale and motivation. The quality of healthcare in the rural and urban areas also differs. While the urban localities have healthcare options from five star medical colleges to small private dispensaries run by trained doctors, the rural areas often are left with the only option of untrained private practitioners. This means that a significant number of the deliveries in these areas are conducted by untrained (traditional) practitioners. This to a large extent affects the quality of maternity care and impacts maternal mortality rates. The following tables and figure show health facilities and health professionals across Cross River State of Nigeria.

s/no	LGA	Type of Health Facility							
		SHF	CHC	PHC	HC	HP	Private	THC	Missoion
1	Abi	1	1	4	5	10	0	0	0
2	Akamkpa	2	0	9	15	10	4	0	0
3	Akpabuyo	1	0	7	11	12	1	0	0
4	Bakassi	0	0	0	3	6	0	0	0
5	Bakwara	0	0	3	0	33	4	0	0
6	Biase	1	0	2	27	1	3	0	0
7	Boki	0	2	10	24	17	5	0	2
8	Calabar 1	1	0	3	2	18	30	1	0
9	Calabar 2	1	0	2	7	16	21	1	0
10	Etung	0	0	8	3	1	0	0	0
11	Ikom	0	1	13	0	12	11	0	1
12	Obanliku	1	0	3	11	24	0	0	1
13	Obubra	2	1	3	14	10	4	0	0
14	Obudu	0	0	3	8	16	5	0	1
15	Odukpani	0	1	6	3	24	1	0	0
16	Ogoja	2	0	8	15	16	13	0	1
17	Yakurr	1	0	9	0	14	8	0	0
18	Yala	2	2	2	26	31	8	0	1

*Source: Cross River State Ministry of Health in Nigeria, 2008.

SFH – Secondary Health Care   HC – Health Centre
CHC – Comprehensive Health Centre   HP – Health Post
PHC – Primary Health Care   THC - Tertiary Health Centre

Table 1: Summary of Health Facilities in Cross River State by LGA

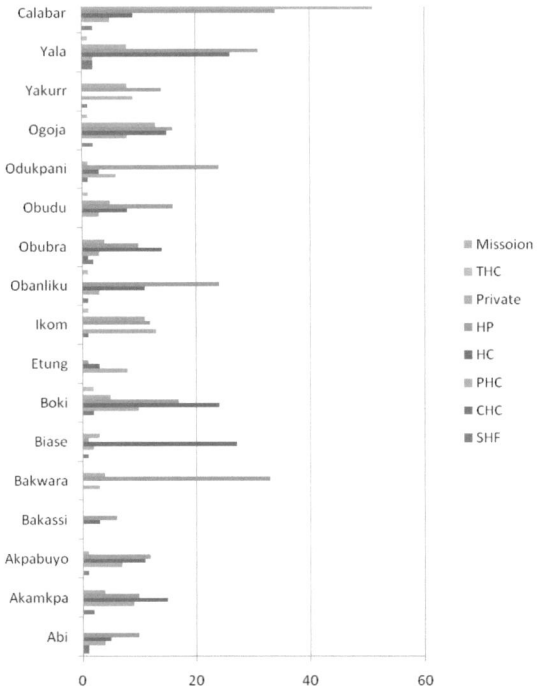

Fig 2: Summary of Health Facilities in Cross River State (Nigeria) by LGA

	LGA	Doctors	Nurses	Pharmacist	Med. Lab. Sc.	Paramedical & others
1	Abi	3	53	0	0	43
2	Akamkpa	8	76	0	2	0
3	Akpabuyo	5	61	0	1	16
4	Bakassi	0	0	0	0	1
5	Bakwara	3	0	0	0	2
6	Biase	6	27	0	1	26
7	Boki	3	10	0	0	5
8	Calabar 1	59	582	8	7	403
9	Calabar 2	22	50	0	0	77
10	Etung	0	0	0	0	2
11	Ikom	10	30	0	1	16
12	Obanliku	5	49	0	1	31
13	Obubra	5	44	0	1	20
14	Obudu	5	55	0	1	10
15	Odukpani	0	5	0	0	0
16	Ogoja	15	136	1	0	69
17	Yakurr	8	63	1	1	30
18	Yala	10	39	0	2	8

Table 2: Summary of health service professionals in cross river state of Nigeria.

4

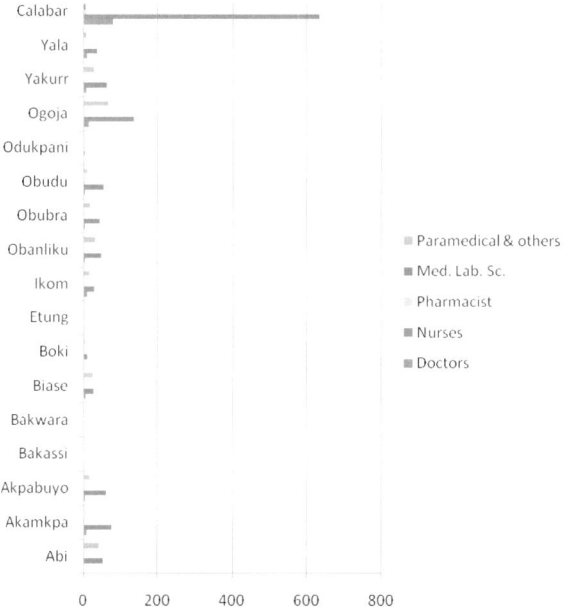

Fig 3: Summary of health service professionals in cross river state of Nigeria

c) Cost of healthcare

Providing healthcare services to the poor at a reasonable cost requires a significant amount of subsidy, either through government or non-government source.

Components of ICT

ICT is a collection of technologies and applications which enable electronic processing, storing and transfer of information to a wide variety of users or clients.[9] These technologies and applications are further broadly classified into three categories on the basis of their use, viz. (1) computing; (2) communication; and (3) internet – enabled communication and computing.[10]

Application of ICT

Information and communication technology has a very important role to play in facilitating quality healthcare to the rural poor in a cost effective manner. In an age of high-tech medical care, those excluded from the mainstream healthcare service could be provided with the benefits of medical professionals through the use of an appropriate ICT kiosk. This needs a joint commitment from both private and public sector.

Telemedicine is used as a means to provide health access to people in the rural community through the use of various kiosks. However, this has not become popular among the rural poor because of inadequate know-how on the use of various kiosks. In a situation where large-scale technology illiteracy exists, it is important to promote appropriate technology kiosks that would be easy for the poor to use. Use of telephones could be a starting point for rural areas. Even operation of a telephone is complicated for many living in rural areas.

Tele-clinics

Tele-clinic is a telephone enabled closed network of rural people, trained health workers and medical professionals. This network enables communication between doctor and a patient in a remote rural village with the help of a telephone. A trained health worker facilitates the communication between a doctor and a patient through a phone provided by government owned telecommunication agency.

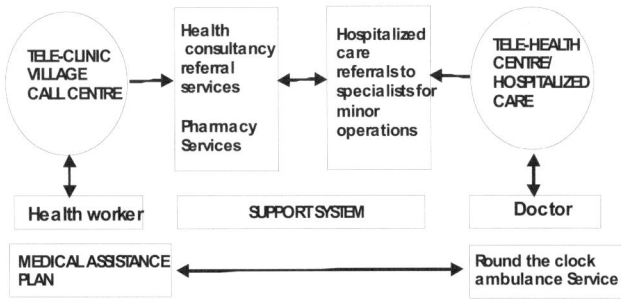

Fig 4: Tele-clinic: ICT solution model

A trained health worker is recruited in all the call centres. These call centres provide services like primary healthcare, ambulance service, telephone consultation, emergency drugs and so on. One call centre covers three to five surrounding villages. Each of the tele-health centres situated in zones is linked via VSAT (fig 6), so that audio and visual communication (teleconferencing) is possible. In this way professional assistance can easily be rendered by a major/ specialised physician in the medical area in question.

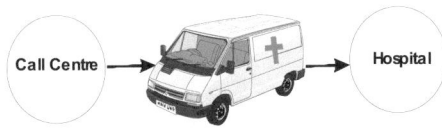

Fig 5: Ambulance service

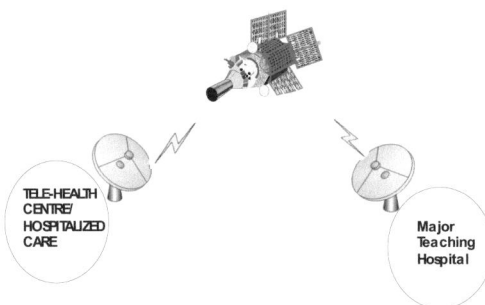

Fig 6: Teleconferencing Infrastructure

Tele-clinic components

1. **Village Call Centres**: Call centres are a very important component of the Tele-clinic. These centres are established in the villages where Tele-clinic project is initiated. A trained health worker mans the call centres. The health worker is called Tele-health Worker (THW), who is provided with a

telephone, basic diagnostic equipments and emergency drugs. Call centres provide the following main services:

a) Telephone consultation with a doctor at the Hospital
b) Emergency drugs
c) Clinical support through nurse-run-clinics
d) Health awareness through periodical campaigns

2. **Ambulance Service**: A round the clock ambulance service is provided by the Tele-clinic Project to provide access to the hospitals. A separate phone number is given to access the ambulance and this service is available any time of the day or night. Further, this service could be used to visit any hospital in the town at times of emergency.

3. **Medical Assistance Plan (MAP)**: Medical assistance plan is similar to a health insurance and is an important component of Tele-clinic Project. This can be covered by the individuals, government or non-governmental agencies.

Levels of treatment
Tele-clinic uses a three tier healthcare service through use of Information and Communication Technology.

a) Call Centre level – primary care - manned by a health worker:
b) Weekly referral clinics at Call Centre Level – Manned by nurse & laboratory technician
c) Hospital level – secondary care

At all these levels the consultation of a qualified practitioner / a specialist is important. All treatments are provided after specialist consultation over phone or by teleconferencing, except in case of causalities where health worker administer emergency drugs / refer the patient to the hospital.

Value addition to rural healthcare

- Promotion of good practices in healthcare in rural areas: There will be a remarkable change in the practices related to healthcare in the villages after the introduction of Tele-clinics. Healthcare will be available to the poor.
- Improved access to specialists through a telecommunication network.
- Improved access to hospitals through a round the clock ambulance service.
- Professional isolation gap is bridged.

Conclusions
ICT is not sufficient to ensure improvement in the well-being of rural dwellers. Application of ICT should be supplemented with appropriate social protection policies which would enable the poor to actually benefit from information/knowledge. Practicing information is not just a function of availability of options but depends on the supplementary policies that enable practicing in real life situations. [11]
Not only the government, the private sector should also be socially responsible. The IT companies and educational institutions should respond to the social cause through developing rural friendly communication kiosks and rendering technology education in rural areas.

Civil society institutions should take up the job of building the capacities of the traditional actors such as untrained health workers, private practitioners, traditional birth attendants and other health workers within the community apart from their role of building partnerships. The Public Health Network through technology should include these actors who are working at the very local level. Linking them with qualified medical practitioners could bring change in overall health condition of the poor in rural areas. ICT could be also used in facilitating a continuing medical education to the practitioners in the rural localities. They are an important part of the 'rural healthcare system'. However, the practices will need to be standardised through adequate trainings and regulation.

The call centres could also perform as 'knowledge banks'. This would be a two-way knowledge bank that gathers tacit knowledge from rural communities and promotes current information on various issues related to rural livelihood. The information on product markets, labour markets, commerce, etc. also could be made available through call centres, which could affect the livelihood of the poor living in the rural areas. The centre could be transformed as 'knowledge centres', which would have information on a range of human development aspects from health, education to livelihood.

Recommendation
Finally, there is ample potential for effective use of ICT in healthcare and initiatives are promising. However, much still remains to be done. Several future trends of great importance are:
* Converging of media and tools for communication
* Increased web-based storage of medical information
* Cheaper and improved connectivity for rural communities

• Increased recognition by governments of the importance of the use of ICT in rural development
• Increased tailor-made, quality healthcare information services.

REFERENCES

1. Long, K.A. The Concept of Health. Rural Nursing; 1993;28:123-130.

2. S. Denise, "The case for e-health,"2003, [online] Available at: http://www.eipa.nl/Publications/Summaries/ 03/2003_E_01.pdf.

3. S. Y. Kwankam, "What E- Health can offer," Bulletin of World Health Organ, vol. 82, no.10, Ge nebra Oct. 2004.

4. J. K. H. Tan, Health Management information Systems; Methods and practical Applications. 2001

5. Peter W Gething et al, Improving Imperfect Data from Health Management Information Systems in Africa Using Space–Time Geostatistics. PLoS Med. 2006 June; 3(6): e271. Published online 2006 June 6. doi:10.1371/journal.pmed.0030271.

6. G. Eysenbach and T. L. Diepgen. "The role of e-health and consumer health informatics for evidence-based patient choice in the 21st century". Clinics in Dermatology, vol. 19, no. 1, pp. 11–17, 2001.

7. M. McMullan." Patients using the Internet to obtain health information: How this affects the patient–health professional relationship". Patient Education and Counselling, vol. 63, no. 1–2, pp. 24–28, Oct. 2006.

8. Hill, K., C. AbouZahr, and T. Wardlaw. 2001. "Estimates of Maternal Mortality for 1995." Bulletin of the World Health Organization 79 (3): 182-193.

9. Cohen G., Salomon I. & Nijkamp P. 2002. Information–communications technologies (ICT) and transport: does knowledge underpin policy? Telecommunications Policy Volume 26, Issues 1-2 , February-March 2002, Pages 31-52.

10. Quibria M.G., Ahmed N. S., Tschang T. & Reyes-Macasaquit M. 2003.Digital divide: determinants and policies with special reference to Asia. Journal of Asian Economics, Volume 13, Issue 6, January 2003, Pages 811-825.

11. Foros Q., Kind H.J. & Sand J.Y.2005. Do internet incumbents choose low interconnection quality? Information Economics and Policy. Volume 17, Issue 2 , March 2005, Pages 149-164

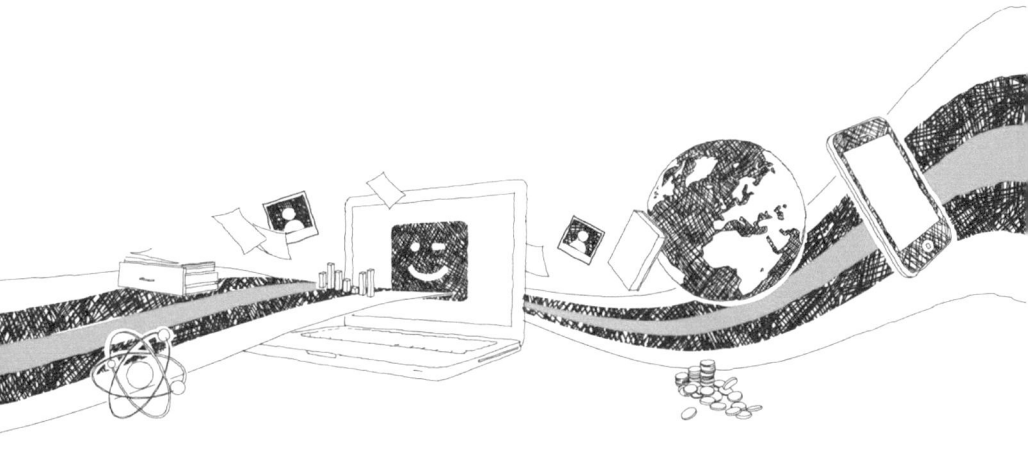
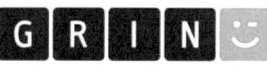